MW01674139

N. A.

HERBAL DISPENSATORY

The Native American Herbal Medicine to Discover the Secrets and Forgotten Practices

Omar Nazir

Table of Contents

Introduction

For decades, Native American herbal medicines have been used to treat chronic diseases and cure diverse health problems. Native Americans depended on the many plants that flourished near their homes, as they have no access to physicians or hospitals. Most of this knowledge has been forgotten; there are, however, some that continue to record the remaining recipes. Native American herbal medicines are still being used to treat numerous illnesses today. However, before trying any herbal cure, you need to study the particular remedy and speak to your health care provider. Native Americans were as vulnerable as anybody else to respiratory problems. Teas derived from natural ingredients or blends of these ingredients were used to treat allergies, coughs and colds. To loosen and remove phlegm, they treated asthma with skunk cabbage. For bronchitis, pneumonia, and other respiratory ailments, the pleurisy root was used. It is also an exceptional cure for these diseases. Wormwood has also been prescribed for multiple bronchitis conditions. For the discomfort of colds and flu, Sage was used. The tribes used the boneset to cure coughs and colds. To treat the cold, a similar aspen tea was prepared from the Aspen tree's inner bark.

For the same reason, Wild Cherry tea, produced from the bark of the Wild Cherry Tree, was also made into tea. Likewise, as a cough syrup, sarsaparilla was mixed with the sweet flag. Rabbit tobacco and Bloodroot were similarly used to relieve different effects of cold, cough and flu. To get relief from back pain, they used arnica as a rub or a poultice. Also, horsemint tea was drunk to deal with back pains. Under the harsh conditions under which many tribes existed, diarrhea may easily cause dehydration. When stomach problems arose, these Native American herbal medicines were used. Unless otherwise noted, these treatments were used in tea form.

Diarrhea

- Black cherry root
- Dogwood bark tea is used as enemas.
- Black Raspberry root
- Black cherry fruit was fermented naturally for up to a year. Finally, the juice was used to cure dysentery.

Other Digestive Disorders

- Dandelion roots were used to treat urinary tract problems and heartburn.
- Yellow Root was used as a cure for stomach related issues.
- Sage was used to treat stomach problems.
- Juniper was used to cure urinary tract infections.
- Juniper was also used to treat diarrhea.
- Elder was used as a laxative.

To get relief from menstrual cramps, provide ease in childbirth, remedy hormonal imbalances, and fix libido disorders, Wild Yam root was used very effectively. They used sage in a particular manner to manage irregular menstruation, childbirth-related complications and bleeding.

Passion Flower was used for:

- Tension
- Insomnia
- Earache

They used willow to treat:

- Pain
- Fever
- Headache

Purple Coneflower was used to cure:

- Snakebite
- Insect bites
- Toothaches

They used Black Cohosh to manage and treat the following issues:

- Female hormones
- Tinnitus
- Sciatica

- Arthritis
- Cough
- Headaches

Skullcap was used to treat:

- Restless leg
- Nervous tension
- Insomnia

The herbal medicines that the Native Americans used to cure many diseases are still being grown, gathered and produced by many Native Americans. Many of the popular natural medicines you find are before Native American treatments in your local health food store. Many of those herbs used by the Native Americans were given for their diseases to early settlers. For centuries, these herbs have been used, and many were in traditional medicinal usage before the advent of mainstream medicines. Any of the choices for capsules and tinctures we have were not available to Native Americans. It's more than probable that much of their herbal medicines were made into teas. Modern types of these herbs have the same function and work as tea in many cases. This book contains several remedies and preparation techniques to help you naturally treat different sicknesses.

Native American Medicine

Through a powerful oral tradition, Native Americans' generations have obtained medical information over the past 40,000 years. The interconnection between humanity, ecology, and the spiritual realm is emphasized by indigenous medical philosophy. A person of medicine studies the relationships of the patient with other individuals, the individual's physical well-being, and establishes a holistic approach for healing. A combination of therapies and experiences are used to treat and cure the patient. These may include herbs, ceremony, music, prayer and sweating.

To cure cardiovascular disorders and many other cancers and diseases, black cohosh, a traditional medicinal herb, was used. The effectiveness of Native American medical therapies is now accepted by western medicine. Traditional and new medicines are not inherently mutually exclusive. Thus they can be used in concert with each other. Any of the plants used by Native American physicians can now be found in commercial stores around the country. They include black cohosh that is used to treat cardiovascular issues. Similarly, Echinacea is used to cure infections.

Native American Medicine History

Native American medicine relates to over 500 nations' combined clinical practices. Native medicine is almost forty thousand years old. The particular activities differed between tribes, but everything is based on the universal idea that man is an integral part of nature and that a matter of balance is health. When interrelationships are valued, nurtured and sustained in harmony, the natural world then moves as a consequence. The natural world cannot be seen by the mind and does not engage in science directly and intuitively. Much like a human being's inner life cannot be determined, nature has persuasive forces that need to be incorporated for balance. Just now has reporting started and has been limited to findings, so it is incomplete. Native medicine values all life and is not just a body of science or methodology that is scholarly. For fear of exploitation, Native American elders typically do not disclose their knowledge.

The balance between the inner life and open actions is tackled in Native American medicine. They all take into account the body, mind, soul, thoughts, social circle and lifestyle. The choice and desires of a patient are often respected to establish harmony. Bodywork, naturopathy, bone setting, midwifery, hydrotherapy, botanical, and nutritional medicine can be included in every Native American healer's strategy. Often used are ceremonial and ritual medicines. Many of this has been forgotten as only by living practitioners has this undocumented living practice survived. More Native Americans have been involved in protecting their culture, and Native American medicine today is as fluid as ever with this effort.

1.1 The Treatment approach

Native American medicine is a complete framework that balances every sphere of one's life, including lifestyle and social interactions with one inner world. Native medicine assumes that in the divine realm, the roots of every imbalance lie. In the course of every recovery procedure, spiritual approaches are vital. Including fees and rates, clinical approaches are often clearly and uniquely tailored for the patient. They require, as part of the healing method, the process of fee negotiation. The Healing Elder seems to have the most healing strength, and the elder practitioner loses his prestige as a powerful healer when treatment fails. The person in need of healing makes a proposition to the doctor of medicine and waits to see if it is approved. Face-to-face, they rarely negotiate. The customer leaves the bid outside the healer's door, and if it remains there till the morning, it means that it has not been approved, and one can go somewhere. Once they understand, therapy will, for example, start with a behavioral prescription, a pledge, a selfless act, genuine repentance, or scaling a holy mountain. Techniques include self-inquiry and discovery to ascertain whether there is a need for a dietary improvement, prayer, herbs, massage, a sweat lodge ritual or a vision quest.

1.2 Theories

The main objective is to alter the patient's comprehension of the world through a healthier self-concept, increased acceptance of others and behavior adjustments. The healer's goal is not only to treat sickness but to change the patient's overall approach towards life and the world around him. Native American medicine combines science as well as spirit with the onset of new technology. They mostly use herbal interventions and pharmaceuticals. We can explain this by narrating a Native American story on the use of herbal medicine. Barb, a wife, mother and lawyer, is still fighting breast cancer. She did what she could normally do, and the cancer continued to spread despite all her efforts. She met with an Indian elder named Big Nose in a sweat lodge. He wanted to understand what she was doing or what hadn't changed in her life. Deep inside, as a mother-wife and lawyer, she thought she was a loser, and now she's healing herself. It was the pessimistic self-talk that needed to end, Big Nose told her. Barb decided to let go of her arrogant thought that she would be cured and started to enjoy the moment with her family due to this relationship. There is another story that talks of a woman who had had extreme arthritis. She was desperately looking for the right healer. To facilitate recovery, medicine men go further and beyond the current problem and understand radical improvement is often required. The shifts are primary, and herbs are secondary, along with massage and prayer. Right relationships, the correction of relationships with oneself, families, members of the society and the spiritual environment are all effects of disruption of relationships and disease development.

Training

Native American healers, through apprenticeships, educate their students. For preparation, several weeks of testing the purpose and dedication of a student are vital. An apprentice gains patience and respect and acquires knowledge. Native medicine is still an oral tradition. It cannot be taught in an academic setting. Students may learn the skills required only by experience, and only when the patient is ready does the older instructor encourage them to begin a medical practice.

The Main Role of Ceremonies

A crucial aspect of traditional aboriginal healing is the ritual. Due to the close relationship between physical & spiritual well-being, body and soul should heal together. Popular healing rituals encourage well-being by representing ancestral concepts of the world, creator, and spirit. Prayer, drumming, chants, poems, legends & the use of several religious artifacts may be part of them. Wherever an ill person requires healing, healers can perform ceremonies, but the ceremonies are sometimes performed in sacred places. The special buildings are also mentioned as the Medicine Lodges for healing. Traditional healing rituals are considered holy wherever they take place & are only performed by the native healers & local spiritual facilitators. The Non-Natives can take part only by invitation. Native powwows, on the other hand, have grown today into most social and cultural activities that include indigenous music, singing, drumming, regalia, and food. Most powwows welcome all persons.

The Medicine Wheel and the Four Directions

Medicine Wheel, also referred to as the Holy Hoop, has been used for health and healing by thousands of diverse Native American tribes. Also, Father Heaven, Spirit Tree, and Mother Earth represent the Four Paths, symbolizing the dimensions of well-being and life cycles. There are several different shapes that Medicine Wheel could take. It could be artwork, or a real structure on the ground, such as an artifact or painting. Over the past few decades, hundreds of thousands, even, of the medicine wheels that have been constructed on tribal lands in North America. Movement is circular in Medicine Wheel & in the Native American formalities, & typically in the direction of the clock, or the direction is sun-wise. It tends to sync with nature's powers, like gravity & sun's rising & setting.

1.3 Meanings of the Four Directions

Medicine Wheel is viewed differently by various tribes. Usually, each of the Four Directions (West, East, North and South) is represented by a distinctive hue, such as red, black, yellow, & white, representing human races for some. The Directions may also indicate:

- **Stages of life:** the birth, youth, adulthood (or elder) and death
- **Element of the nature:** sun (or fire), water, earth and air
- **Animals:** Bear, Eagle, Buffalo, Wolf, & many more
- **Seasons of the year:** spring, summer, winter, fall

- **Aspects of life:** spiritual, emotional, intellectual, physical
- **Ceremonial plants:** sweet grass, tobacco,cedar, sage

1.4 Healing Plants

For a broad range of medical uses, Alaska Native, Native American & healers of Native Hawaiian all have a long tradition of using the native or indigenous plants. Medicinal plants are as varied as tribes that use them and their uses. Beyond their medical effects, before Western settlement, native plants were the staple of aboriginal people's diet. Today, the indigenous plant is central to current generations' attempts to enhance nutritional wellbeing. "Waianae Diet" & "Pre-Captain Diet Cook" are trying to decrease fat, empty calories, & additives. At the same time they are trying to facilitate a healthier and diet that is balanced by restoring indigenous foods' role.

1.5 Intersections of Traditional and Western Healing

Today, the issue of either depending on conventional native healing practices or pursuing Western medical care is frequently confronted by Native Americans of both groups. The two cultures existed in tandem relatively until recently, with really no intersections between them. However, now, the continuum of health services can be accessed by Native Americans. Within tribal communities, most traditional healers are still practicing independently. To organize treatment for Native American patients, other healers can collaborate with Western-trained foremost care physicians. Some healthcare facilities, often at the same location, provide both conventional and Western medicine. In certain areas, rather than by tribal health centers or hospitals, patients of Native Americans receive conventional healing from inside the local tribal population. In the Upper

Plains Tribes of Lakota and Dakota, & Mandan, Hidatsa, & Arikara, (MHA), tribal member arranges for the services by directly calling nearby healers. Many Western-trained doctors often recommend patients to conventional healers and may sometimes assist a specific patient in coordinating traditional and Western medicine.

Mint and Sage Herbal Remedies

The Mint family's plants resemble with feathers of the birds. Moreover, by observing and comparing them, you can discover that they share the following characteristics:

- Four-Sided Square Stems
- Extremely aromatic (Majority of the mint family plants have a strong aroma)
- Tiny flowers have five united petals (three down, two-up). Together they make upper & lower "lips" which form tubule which is just right for the hummingbirds & butterflies
- Flowers are usually arranged in clusters at leaves' base or end of the spikes
- Nearly 1/2 of the common kitchen's spices are from the mint family

2.1 Mint Family Herbal Medicine

The aromatic essence of the family plants of mint comes from their elevated levels of volatile oils, which also explains for rich flavors & many of the medicinal properties valued in cooking. Although plants of mint family's medicinal actions make a reasonably long list and all of them fall into the categories of four:

- Nervine for complaints affecting the nervous system (depression, anxiety, headaches, dementia, insomnia)
- Digestive for concerns about the digestive system: (gas, indigestion, cramps, colic, nausea)
- Antimicrobials for the infections: (viral, fungal, bacterial)
- Clearing for concerns about the respiratory system (infection, asthma, congestion)

The plants comprise volatile oils, including, but not limited to, thymol, menthol, citronellal, camphor, limonene, carvacrol, & linalool. Aside from antimicrobial behavior, the main action of the volatile oils in our internal organs is to reduce stress and spasm. Our good smell sense is closely associated with the brain's limbic system, regulating feeling and memory. Nerve finishing is activated to transmit signals to the limbic system & to systems that control discomfort in the internal organs when we catch the fragrance of an aromatic plant; as volatile oils reach our blood, muscles that are smooth in airways & circulatory tissues inside the intestines are relaxed, relieving strain & restoring balance. As for nervine effects, feelings of "existing in flow" or sense of equilibrium is mirrored in our mental condition by the relaxed state generated in our internal organs. It is most probable because fresh smells mean a changing atmosphere and behave as a wake-up request, helping us shift from a tense environment to a calmer state. Briefly, the volatile oil is excellent for destroying microorganisms, from microbes and fungi to viruses, concerning the antimicrobial activity of mint family plants. During periods of illness and disease, aromatics were utilized as the strewing herbs inside homes in Middle Ages to fight 'evil,' also known as microorganisms. And as a sinus infection cure, what else could have been more divine than the mint family aromatherapy? The aromatic activity of the plants of the mint family relaxes tissue of the respiratory system & clears the airways, causing congestion to pass out and breathing to flow easily, whether it is a cup of peppermint tea for the nasal congestions, facial steam of thyme for soothing cough, or the hyssop syrup for moving lung congestion.

2.2 The Mint Family Herbal Remedies

Lemon glycerite balm, a bowl of the tabbouleh with the spearmints for lunch, a whiff of lavender essential oil during rush hour traffic, a cup of cool peppermint tea as a midday-afternoon pick-up, calming cup of the catnip tea soon after a meal, or a revitalizing foot soak of lavender essential oil during rush hour traffic, are so many simple ways to incorporate the uplifting, soothing, and tasty essence of mint into your day. Given below are a few quick remedies.

2.3 Peppermint Sun Tea

It is an amazing and excellent recipe for a hot summer day. We have listed below the ingredients that you would require for preparing this Native American herbal recipe:

- Half cup or one cup dried or fresh peppermint leaves.
- Half gallon of tap water.

Given below are the detailed instructions for preparing this Native American herbal recipe. You need to follow these instructions in the given order.

- Put peppermint & water in half a gallon of a glass jar.

- Put in a sunny area for two to eight hours.
- Move to the fridge and let it cool. Enjoy it as a cold drink.

2.4 Tummy Tea

We have listed below the ingredients that you would require for preparing this Native American herbal recipe:

- D Dried chamomile flowers
- catnip leaf, Dried
- lemon balms leaf Dried

Given below are the detailed instructions for preparing this Native American herbal recipe. You need to follow these instructions in the given order.

- Combine equal parts of lemon balm, chamomile and catnip thoroughly in a jar. Then cap & label.
- Then To brew tea, put one tablespoon of the tea blend into eight ounces of water boiled. Then allow it to steep for three to four minutes.
- You can add sweeteners as per your taste, or you may not. Finally enjoy.
- Keep in mind one thing that chamomile will get bitter if it is steeped for a long time.

2.5 Lavender Honey

We have listed below the ingredients that you would require for preparing this Native American herbal recipe:

- Fresh or Dried buds of lavender flower
- Local honey, raw

Given below are the detailed instructions for preparing this Native American herbal recipe. You need to follow these instructions in the given order.

- Fill the jar(either half or quarter) with the flower buds. Next, fill it with honey.
- The air bubbles should be removed by poking with a knife or chopstick. Then mix well.
- Allow the mixture to infuse for a week or month, depends on the preferred strength. You need to taste it occasionally till it's suited perfectly to taste buds.

2.6 Sage and Honey Cough Syrup

The majority of the people do not like to take medicine. Much of the medicine that we need is given by nature. Now we're going to teach you how to make a Cough Syrup of Sage & Honey. It's so easy, but it's effective. Honey is more powerful than any cough medicine from drugstores. Sage is an astringent, anti-bacterial, & anti-inflammatory herb, which makes it perfect for coughs and sore throats. Sage and honey make a delicious cough syrup together, and it's simply that everyone can make one batch. It is such cough syrup that is simple and convenient. As honey is an exceptional preservative, a sample will last indefinitely.

We have listed below the ingredients that you would require for preparing this Native American herbal recipe:

- One cup or two of sage leaves, organic and fresh
- One cup or extra of honey (raw), local preferred
- One clean glass container or jar which can be tightly sealed & can contain at least twelve ounces

Given below are the detailed instructions for preparing this Native American herbal recipe. You need to follow these instructions in the given order.

- Wash & dry the sage properly.
- The leaves should be trimmed from the stems.
- Put sage leaves into the glass jar. Then pour honey over the sage leaves. It would take some while for honey to move between the leave and soak them thoroughly.
- Take a spoon and mix properly. Mix it daily. Allow it to sit for a week.
- Pull out the leaves and squeeze to take out all honey. You can also decant or leave it here & spoon it out as required into a container.
- Administer medicinally for painful throats& coughs in teaspoonfuls, or stir spoonful as a calming tea in a cup of the water (warm) with a lemon's squeeze.

- Tightly pack it and store it in the fridge. As honey is an exceptional preservative, it can last for a long time.

Native American Herbs Preparation

One of the most neglected issues when it comes to emergency preparedness is applying natural herbs and plants for medicinal use. Many people have no idea in the modern world which plants are dangerous and which plants could be used as a medicine, but it wasn't always that way. There is nothing new in using herbs and plants for medicinal use. Under the theory that man is a part of nature, Native Americans utilized them for thousands of years. Also, archaeological findings have shown that man, starting with the ancient Egyptians and Chinese has been using herbs and plants for medicinal purposes since at least 3000 BC. They used herbs and plants to cure oral disorders to stomach aches, headaches, skin rashes and more. It was not until the 1700s and 1800s that scholars and medical practitioners started to study these plants in the Western world. Today, science has progressed to the point that it is extremely rare to include natural ingredients in pharmaceutical medication, even though most of today's drugs derive from elements that exist naturally. Of course, in a survival situation, you certainly won't have any prescription meds. In this situation, the natural herbs and plants that Native Americans used hundreds of years ago would be the next best option. The few that are worth learning about are:

3.1 Blackberries

These are also the same blackberries that have healing qualities that you purchase at the store. The Cherokee tribe will use them, most importantly, to help calm stomach pain. Scientific analysis has revealed today that blackberries are high in antioxidants, which may explain why stomach pain can be minimized. Native Americans used to grind the roots and mix them with honey while consuming blackberries orally. This resulting formula would calm issues with the stomach, alleviate coughs, soothe mouth stores and provide relief to sore throats.

Wild Ginger

Wild ginger was used for medicinal purposes by many Native American tribes. The Cherokee tribe used the plant to facilitate digestion. The tribe used it to help with illnesses such as colic, intestinal bloating and gas, and aches and cramps in the stomach. To remove unnecessary mucus from the lungs, wild ginger was also used. European immigrants who settled in North America had to live without many of the Old Country's comforts of home. However, they discovered a replacement in the rhizomes of an unrelated plant that they called wild or Indian ginger in the case of ginger root (Zingiber officinale) (Asarum canadense). A member of the birthwort family is wild ginger. Around 70 species of low-growing, stem-less perennial herbs with aromatic rhizomes constitute the genus Asarum, mostly native to warm temperate eastern Asia, just a few to North America, and one to Europe.

Uses

Native Americans prepared wild ginger rhizome decoctions and infusions to deal with problems related to menstruation cycles and control irregular heartbeats. To reduce earache, Meskwaki steeped crushed rhizomes and poured the solvent into the ear. There was little denying that early European explorers learned many medical applications from Native Americans. Perhaps an Indian cure was also their teeth powder made from the pulverized bark of black alder, bayberry, and black oak combined with the powdered wild ginger rhizome. However, their use of the candied rhizome and syrup to alleviate flatulence and stomach cramps presumably resulted from similar ginger root use. The "doctrine of signatures" was another Old World influence, according to which the kidney-shaped leaves of wild ginger were a symbol that the plant was intended to be used for curing kidney disorders. Other wild ginger folk uses involved relieving fevers by triggering sweating and curing snakebite (hence one name for it, Canada snakeroot).

3.2 Buckbrush

To survive, you need at least one of your kidneys to work properly, and buckbrush is one of the best natural materials to achieve your kidneys good functioning. To treat tumors and cysts, inflammation and sore throats, buckbrush can also be used. This herb was historically used with diuretic properties as a medicinal substance. It has historically been used to promote the efficient functioning of the kidneys. To treat mouth and throat problems, inflammation, and cysts and tumors, members of almost the same plant family have also been utilized. These herbs also address particular health conditions, such as inflamed tonsils, aftercare for miscarriage, hemorrhoids, enlarged spleens and swollen lymph nodes. Its easiest and most effective use is in the form of tea. Boil some water for five to ten minutes and put the roots in it. To receive the full benefits, you may then continue to drink the resulting buckbrush tea.

3.3 Wild Black Cherry, One of the Great North American Herbs

After the logging, wildfires, & other distressed soils like the yard & forest edges, these common trees pop up. They grow rapidly and are vulnerable to the disease, so you're better off learning how to recognize them than humanize them. The Prune trees upto 1 inch in diameter or, for medicine, cut down an entire young tree, scrape off bark& chop up tiny twigs. Then Wait till after the flowering & dry properly before using it in remedies. For acidic, aggravated, spastic coughs & chest symptoms, like wood smoke & wildfires, cherry bark is outstanding. This calms spasms & allows the lungs to open. It acts well as dried plant tincture (to balance bark tannins, add 10 percent glycerine), tea (that is best in tepid or is not relatively boiling water), otherwise processed cold honey or syrups. Often known as chokecherry, wild cherry bark (Prunus serotina, P. virginiana) is one of many herbal remedies containing amygdalin, also known as prunasin, a toxic glycoside contained in seeds of several species of Rosaceae, including peaches, bitter almonds, apricots and loquat, a herb used to alleviate coughing in traditional Chinese medicine (TCM). It is found in blackberry leaves as well. Prunasin's unique property is its ability to prevent the cough reflex, especially in the case of dry cough, which has become one of the most severe long-term complications following influenza in recent years. One of the most successful therapies for asthma, bronchitis and whooping cough that has spread through the US's sectors in recent months is a tea of wild cherry bark and coltsfoot.

Uses

Although herbalists promote the use of wild cherry bark as a sovereign cure for coughs in tea and alcoholic tincture extracts, a misunderstanding occurs when writers describing edible plants are likely to highlight the possible toxic properties of wild cherry. Thus, this flower, in particular arrives with significant mixed messages for the herbalist and user to wade through. There is a scenario in which the adage "the poison is in the dose" remains true. It is possible to safely use wild cherry inner bark.

Historical and Modern Use of Wild Cherry

Native American settlers first learned the medicinal uses of wild cherry bark throughout the United States. In reality, Meriwether Lewis was treated with a twig tea of wild cherry bark on his famous expedition for a severe gastrointestinal illness. Its uses as a general GI tonic, a remedy for diarrhea and sore throat, coughs and colds, as a purgative and applied topically to avoid bleeding, native individuals are on record. Many cautions about its use for pregnant mothers and children under two years of age. Nevertheless, Native Americans employed wild cherry to ease labor pains and gave it to nursing mothers who "drank the tea to pass on the medicinal effects to their infants." From 1820 to 1970, wild cherry bark was mentioned as an official in the US Pharmacopeia, arguably a more enlightened time before Big Pharma systematically established itself. To facilitate rapid recovery, herbalists typically prescribe heroic doses of herbs, especially in acute circumstances. An exception will be this herb. The tea is usually prepared by steeping two tsps of wild cherry bark in one cup of boiling water for ten minutes; it will be safe to drink roughly 3 cups every day. It will also be perfect for anywhere from thirty to sixty drops three times every day of the tincture. Besides being a cough inhibitor, wild cherry bark has numerous other applications. It is used to avoid bleeding, diarrhea and hemorrhoids, for sore throats, colds, and as an astringent. It can also be used to treat jaundice and as a digestive stimulant. The same properties that relax dry, irritable coughs are also useful for anxious palpitations, such that wild cherry bark serves the circulatory and nervous systems as a moderate sedative and other mucosal surfaces, including those of the gastrointestinal and urinary tracts. Bark tea fomentations may be used externally to alleviate pain and facilitate the curing of injury and burn caused by inflammation.

Herbalists also recommend an ointment as a remedy for hemorrhoids and wounds.

Last but not least, as an eyewash for inflamed skin, the wild cherry bark's anti-inflammatory properties are especially effective. Wild cherry bark has been commonly used in formula for people of all ages, often in tea or syrup for cough and upper respiratory disease, for more than 30 years. People with asthma and chronic emphysema can make tea from a handful of equivalent portions of the following dried herbs simmered in a quart of water for 20 minutes:

- Wild cherry bark
- A quarter part lobelia herb
- Several slices of raw ginger
- Coltsfoot
- Comfrey root
- Elecampane
- Yerba santa

Effective preparation

Wild cherry bark is safe and very powerful. Double water percolation is a common and effective cherry bark syrup preparation. In a second cone filled with good old-fashioned sugar, the first percolation drips water through the cone (use organic if it makes you feel better). You are left with a sweet almond tasting syrup by the time it stops pouring, which masks the bitterness of the cherry bark. It may be used for children and adults as a respiratory antispasmodic and anti-tussive, expectorant, and to relieve throat pain. It has served well with pertussis, a tickle in the throat, dry hacking coughs, chest tension, and moderate wheezing that accompanies a respiratory infection.

Marshmallow Leaf and Root

Whenever the lungs and respiratory system are dry or irritated, mallows are the ultimate moisturizing herbs as they are calming & slimy & useful. Meadow environment or the garden pampered beds with lush, mildly moist soil & partial or full sun are the right growth conditions for Mallows. In a variety of habitats, wild mallows flourish. Once you discover its happy spot, it is easy to cultivate; it should be harvested earlier in the season before the descent of Japan's hungry beetles. The marshmallow root produces the most important slime. They are in abundance, and leaves are not difficult to harvest. Feel free to get the flowers included. The calming mucilage contains the finest water extracts: cold infusions, syrup, tea, broth. The taste is moderate and mildly sweet, and more herbal & drying the herbs are excellent in recipes. Avoid the alcohol, except maybe for preservation in limited amounts.

It is possible to showcase its ability to support the respiratory system, which happens to be amongst the biggest properties of Marshmallow Root. It is an outstanding anti-inflammatory as well. This herbaceous perennial plant belongs to the family of mallows. While it belongs to the same genus as the hollyhocks, it appears to be much larger. All have observed the delicate and hairy leaves at least once. Its flowers are white and red with a very thick root. These roots are potent because they produce massive quantities of mucilage. If you want to keep it, you can use its flowers, leaves and stems, which have the same properties as the root. It is beneficial for treating bronchitis, cough, and it is ideal for relieving toothache and mouth sores. Native Americans used this plant to treat wounds and snakebites.

Natural Benefits

For an incredibly long time, herbal remedies have been around. Years before western medicine was around, predecessors of all civilizations used herbal medicines. Few herbals, including marshmallow root, have just as many values, advantages, and medical uses. This is a herbal remedy that is safe and perfect. For example, it may be used as a balm and a digestive aid because of its therapeutic feature. Plus, it can assist with breathing and skin conditions by applying it externally. Using the marshmallow balm for cough and mucus is the normal approach. This will soften the alveoli as soon as you try it, and you will feel a lot better. It is not to mention that expelling mucus and coping with asthma and bronchitis is a wonderful support function of this herb. It is the best combination for treating cystitis and other urinary tract disorders if you blend a marshmallow infused with corn silk. Swallowing this plant will help you enhance renal transit rapidly and ease any existing tension in the kidneys. It is beneficial to apply marshmallow as a poultice for all sorts of skin conditions to treat burns and bad wounds. Plus, in a rich infusion, marshmallow flowers will help you minimize inflammation. Only make sure that you apply it to the affected area. It's almost hard to beat its multiple therapeutic properties; you can't argue it's a one-of-a-kind treat.

- Splendid for treating respiratory illness
- Gives excellent results for urinary tract issues
- Handy first aid for burns and wounds

Revolutionary American Manufacturing

Americans are among the world's biggest customers today. They purchase about 90 million pounds a year of this herb in different forms. These snacks were developed by mixing sugar, egg whites and mallow root sap before modern manufacturing. This has now been largely replaced by corn syrup, starch, gelatin and water. It is useful for lowering the sugar index for people with diabetes before all sugar ingredients are added to the marshmallow root.

Plantain Leaf

In lawns, roads, and perturbed soils, this popular weed can be found. The healthier the soil, the larger it becomes. Plantain is most famously used for insect bites and bee stings as a poultice, but the leaves are also calming and curing when used in lung recipes. In addition to boggy dampness, they relieve irritation and dryness, softly moisturizing while still serving to clean, tighten, and tone the mucus covering. They could also provide antimicrobial activity. Consider this for syrups and tea. It has a moderate, friendly and lightly tannic flavor.

What is Plantain?

A common backyard herb with large leaves is Plantain or Plantago Major. Many people, while it is an extremely useful herb, think of it as a weed. Legend has it found by Alexander the Great and carried back to Europe with him in 327 BCE. It has been referred to by Native Americans as the Whiteman's Foot, as everywhere they go, it appeared to pop up, and it's seen as an invasive, noxious weed in some areas. However, it is a useful little herb. Many civilizations worldwide also used it, and the Saxons considered it one of their nine holy herbs. It was considered an early Christian sign of the faithful's path and is referred to as an aphrodisiac by many cultures today. These leaves are very edible and are sometimes used raw & cooked as greens. The Older leaves also have a better taste, often objectionable, and can be tough and stringy, but can be used for tea making. Plantain has a very high concentration of vitamins C and A and calcium. Native Americans used plantain leaves medicinally to ease the bee stings & bites of insects, avoid the itching caused by poison ivy& more allergic rashes, & facilitate healing of sores& bruises. Plantain tea could even be used as an expectorant and mouthwash to help cure and avoid sores in the mouth. Most recently, plantain has been promoted to avoid smoking, bringing another application to the versatile herb's useful applications. Plantain was used in some cultures of Native Americans as a panacea and for some very great reasons. Also, being antitoxic and anti-inflammatory, many of its active components possess antibacterial and antimicrobial effects. A common remedy for bug & animal bites is the leaves, which can be chewed or shredded. The antibacterial activity helps deter infection & anti-inflammatory helps relieve discomfort, burning & itching. To study the effects on reducing blood sugar, some research is underway.

The Many Uses of Plantain

Plantain leaf can be made into a tea, tincture or infusion. Plantain leaf can also be used internally:

- To help get Cholesterol to healthy Levels
- For Hemorrhoid relief
- To help get relief from Irritable Bowel Syndrome
- To help calm the bowels during Constipation or Diarrhea

- To aid people suffering from Diabetes
- To treat kidney and bladder problems.
- To aid with a Bladder infection, ITIs and similar problems.
- It is safe for children
- It can be used for treating indigestion and ulcers

Plantain Leaf is also very soothing on external inflammation:

- Bites
- Burns
- Cuts
- Yeast
- Stings
- Rashes
- Eczema
- Psoriasis
- Varicose Veins

How to Use Plantain

If your yard grows fresh plantain, you should make sure it has not been sprayed with chemicals or pets and use it in teas or salads with young leaves.

Make a poultice of fresh plantain leaf or bentonite clay with water to form a paste for stings and bites. When applied to the bite or sting, it will quickly take away the discomfort. Chew up a plantain leaf and spit on the bite if you don't have the other ingredients close by. It sounds disgusting, but it relieves the pain tremendously. An injection of strong tea of plantain leaf (dried or fresh) would cool the burn and ease the discomfort when sprayed on a sunburn. This can also aid Poison Ivy rashes and reactions. It would help if you steeped plantain leaves (fresh or dried) in apple cider vinegar for a couple of weeks to produce an even better solution and then strain. The flavored vinegar can very easily alleviate swelling, burning, and skin pain. Indigestion, heartburn or IBS can be soothed with a cup of plantain tea from fresh or dried leaves. It is a source of relief for all sorts of digestive problems. It also helps in treating UTIs, urinary infections or kidney infections.

White Pine

The eastern white pine is a native of North America, growing from Newfoundland to Manitoba and eastern Canada. The resin and needles were believed to have medicinal value by the First Nations. As a soothing ointment, the resin, which has certain antiseptic qualities, was smeared on wounds and boiled up to produce a tonic drink. Rich in vitamin C, the needles provided a tea that helped prevent and cure scurvy. Pine was a common ingredient in many mixtures during the heyday of patent medicines in the late 1800s. Pine has good selling potential and possesses certain antiseptic properties: the strong smell reached blocked sinuses and indicated that a strong remedy must be at work. Beyond the apparent one of providing wood, Eastern white pine also had many non-medicinal applications. First Nations used the resin to seal the seams in canoes; pine resins eventually became the basis of consumer goods like pitch and turpentine. The eastern white pine is mainly harvested for its lumber and pulp. The oils used for medicinal purposes are a by-product.

Worldwide, there are over one hundred species of pine, and most have medicinal uses. The needles, inner bark, and resin have been used by civilizations worldwide for similar ailments. Internally, for coughs, colds, asthma, and urinary tract and sinus diseases, pine is a typical treatment. Topically, pine is used in arthritic disorders to combat skin diseases and to lessen joint inflammation. About twenty species of pine have been used in a similar medicinal manner by native communities throughout the continent, including the Chippewa, Cherokee, Iroquois, Apache, Hopi and numerous other groups.

Medicinal Use of Pine Needles

The fresh needles and buds collected in the springtime are called "pine tops." They are boiled in water, and for fevers, coughs, and colds, the tea is consumed. The needles are also used for their diuretic features, helping to improve urination. Pine-top tea, particularly given the abundance of pines in the area, is one of the most valuable historical medicines of the rural south-eastern United States. Famed Alabama herbalist Tommie Bass uses the needles in a steam inhalation to break up the lungs' tenacious phlegm.

For this reason, you may mix pine tops with sprigs of fresh thyme and bee balm. Pine induces relaxation by its relaxing expectorant, antimicrobial, & anti-inflammatory characteristics in sinus and lung congestion. Vitamin C is also in the fresh, younger needles. Try mixing peppermint and catnip as a tea with pine needles, which can be sipped to soothe cold symptoms during the day. For the entire household, this mixture is a healthy cure.

- Mighty Pine Tea

- 1-quart water
- A fistful of pine needle tops (about five to seven branch tips; fresh or dried)
- One and a half tbsp dried peppermint
- One tbsp dried catnip

For twenty minutes, boil the pine needle tops in water. Turn the heat off, and the peppermint and catnip are inserted. Cover and allow to steep for an extra twenty minutes. If needed, strain and add honey. While hot, sip on the tea, reheating each cup during the day as needed. Adults can consume three cups a day. The dosages for children should be lowered proportionally.

Pine Bark

The inner bark contains more resin than the needles and is more astringent. It has traditionally been used for muscular aches and pains as an antimicrobial wash and poultice and infused into bathwater. It is sometimes boiled in water and consumed for coughs and colds as a cure. The knotty pine wood of many pine types is mixed into wine in Traditional Chinese Medicine and then used topically for joint pain.

Pine Resin

There are numerous local first-aid applications of the resin, also called pitch. It is used as an antimicrobial dressing for wounds and to extract splinters. Pine resin has been used internally as a strong expectorant in minute quantities. You can use pine pitch to pull out splinters, glass, and the contaminants left from toxic bug bites prepared as a salve. Pine resin salve is effective in reducing muscle aches and inflammation of the joints.

Pine Pitch Band-Aids: Forest First-Aid

Take a semi-hard but pliable piece of pitch and form it over the affected region into a flat bandage. While also being anti-inflammatory and antimicrobial, this basic first-aid has excellent drawing ability. Cover it and leave it on overnight with a Band-Aid or clean bandage.

- Pine Pitch Salve
- One part clean pine pitch
- Two parts extra-virgin olive oil
- Grated beeswax beads

Melt the olive oil pitch using a double boiler (1 part pitch to 2 parts olive oil, by volume) until it is completely melted (it's okay if a little resin stays solid). Add the grated beeswax (one-part beeswax per four parts of the combined pitch and liquid oil). Before inserting lids, pour into jars and leave to cool.

Safety & Contraindications

In pregnancy, should not use pine needles and prevent the long-term internal use of bark. With long-term use of heavy doses or with sensitive individuals, the pine needles and pine bark may cause kidney irritation. But in minute doses under the supervision of a certified herbalist, you can use pine resin internally. You should be confident that you have identified pine correctly, and it's not a look-alike or a sound-alike.

Tobacco

There are more than 60 species of tobacco, officially called Nicotiana, that are mostly indigenous to Australia and America. For social, religious, ceremonial purposes and medicinal remedies, plants had also assumed greater importance in Native American culture. Leaves have long been used to remedy boils, poison, skin conditions, measles, vertigo, and to cure mosquitoes and snakebites to prevent nausea, colic, worms, kidney problems, fever, colic, convulsions, toothache. Tobacco and other plant mixtures are grown or harvested and used for ceremonial or medicinal purposes by American Indians, and Alaska Natives are traditional tobacco. For centuries, traditional tobacco has been used as a medicine with cultural and theological significance by American Indian nations. Many tribes preserve the teachings and legends about the roots of tobacco. These teachings deal with tobacco in its simplest form, known today as the Nicotiana rustica tobacco plant, and can contain other indigenous plants' mixtures. The traditional preparation and use of tobacco differ across tribes and territories, with traditional tobacco not widely used by Alaskan natives. These variations are due to the many distinct teachings of the North American Tribes. The functions of cultivating, processing, and preparing conventional tobacco in certain communities are held by unique classes of individuals who use traditional methods to prepare tobacco for a particular use. The significance of maintaining a positive attitude and thoughts even when working with traditional tobacco is one common teaching. Traditional tobacco is a medicine that may be used to promote emotional, physical, spiritual and community well-being in a prescribed manner. A traditional tobacco gift is a sign of respect and might even be offered when requesting assistance, guidance, or protection. In herbal medicine, traditional tobacco is often used specifically for curing. It can be burnt or smoked in a pip, but the smoke is normally not inhaled. The smoke from burning tobacco has the function of bringing thoughts and prayers to the divine world or the

Creator in certain teachings. Traditional tobacco is not linked with tolerance and adverse health effects when used properly. In the planning and usage of conventional tobacco, the care and reverence involved are part of centuries of practice that ties today's children, adults, and elders with those who existed years ago. Today and for future years to come, continued use of traditional tobacco promotes a decent life and a healthy society.

3.4 Cattail

Cattail is more like a prevention therapy than an active drug. Except for the seeds and the leaves, any part of the plant can be consumed. For open wounds such as bruises, abrasions, and scrapes, Cattail is best used as an antiseptic. The Cattail's root may be simply broken open and brought into close contact with the open wound, then tied with a rope or paracord. Also, for this same therapeutic purpose, cattail ash may be used.

Simply put it into close contact with the wound that is open. Currently, the legend says that, with a little support from the humble Cattail, the US was on the brink of winning World War 2. More edible starch than almost any other green plant is produced by Cattail (starch per acre). From this point of view, rice, potatoes, yams, or taros are less nutritious than Cattail. Lichen is the only plant capable of beating cattails in terms of carbs per acre (starch is the essential carbohydrate), although this is not a green plant. An acre of cattails can, however, yield 6.5K pounds of flour annually on average.

Health benefits of Cattail

Cattail is one of the plants that are cultivated worldwide that are good and nutrient-rich. Some of the common health benefits of cattail consumption are described in detail below:

Improves digestion

Cattail consists of a good amount of soluble and insoluble fiber necessary for the digestive system's proper functioning. Soluble fibers counter cholesterol accumulation and insoluble fiber enables waste to pass out of the environment. This adds to lower chances of hemorrhoids or even constipation. So use cattail in your diet to eliminate all of the issues associated with digestion.

Calorie rich

If you are undernourished and want to add some weight, the easiest way is to pair Cattails' rich diet with a wholesome dinner. The weight gain process is facilitated because the cattail is high in nutrients and calories. It is also one of the beneficial choices for underweight individuals to achieve the required body weight.

Skin Health

Cattail consists of immense quantities of nutrients and organic compounds, which primarily promotes its ability to cure boils, sores, lessen the occurrence of scars, and add to its effect on the skin. Topically, cattail jelly should be used for mosquito bites, but the flour also has an anti-inflammatory ability that reduces some affected discomfort and severity.

Hypertension

Adrenal glands are given sufficient assistance to minimize stress levels due to Cattail's protein and carbohydrate content. It tends to increase the rate of metabolism and hence lowers stress.

Diabetes

Phytochemicals are needed for insulin absorption. Your system can combat diabetes mellitus, which is non-insulin-dependent, by taking Cattail daily. So eating Cattail daily to fight diabetes is fruitful.

Cancer Prevention

However, this field of study is somewhat new and somewhat contentious, but research is underway on cattails' potential to prevent cancer. Chinese researchers are leading a promising new field of study, but its antioxidant effects on cancer cells are promising.

Atherosclerosis

Because of the presence of vitamin C, carotenoids and bioflavonoids, the intake of Cattail decreases LDL. These components ensure that coronary disease complications are minimized, and the LDL is cleaned out of the system. Apart from that, the absorption of cholesterol is also decreased. This suggests a lowered chance of developing atherosclerosis.

Cardio tonic and lipid-lowering effects

There is a certain composition of compounds in the Cattail, which reduces the lipids in the body and dilates the coronary artery. It is used to treat coronary conditions such as angina, hyperlipidemia, etc. It is also used for dissolving stasis. It tends to decrease lipid accumulation on the artery walls. Hence, the occurrence of heart failure is reduced.

Antiseptic Application

Cattail is famous because of its natural antiseptic quality, which has come in handy for various cultures for centuries. In wounds and other parts of the body where foreign agents, bacteria, or microbes could harm our system, the jelly-like compounds you will find between young leaves are used. This same jelly is regarded as a potent analgesic from the cattail plant, which can be eaten or applied topically to alleviate discomfort and inflammation.

Steady increase in energy

As we all know, a rich source of energy is carbohydrates. There is a decent amount of starch content in Cattail. It means that it has the potential to give you higher energy levels and even replenish energy levels from time to time if they are insufficient. The breakdown is very slow because Cattail is made up of complex carbohydrates, which means you will have all the energy you need for the day.

Slow Bleeding

Different portions of the Cattail have coagulant properties, which ensures they slow down blood supply and prevent anemia. If you are injured, this can be effective, but also if you suffer from excessive menstrual bleeding, reducing the severity. But for patients who still have moderately poor circulation, it is potentially harmful because it essentially slows blood down while also stimulating the skin's coagulant response.

How to Eat

- Several parts of the herb, including dormant sprouts on the leaves' roots and bases, ripe pollen, the stem and starchy roots, are edible.
- Raw or cooked roots are edible.
- They can be boiled and eaten similar to potatoes or macerated to create sweet syrup and then boiled.

- Roots may also be dried or ground into a powder and subsequently used or added to cereal flours as a thickener in soups, etc., and this protein-rich powder is used to produce cookies, etc.

Young shoots are eaten raw or cooked during the spring.

The base of the mature stem can also be consumed both raw or cooked.

It is often edible raw, fried or prepared in a soup, the tender, young flowering stem.

Pollen is edible, raw, cooked or refined into a rich in protein additive used in the processing of bread, porridge, etc.

Tiny seeds can be roasted or fried, and edible oil can be extracted from the seeds.

3.5 Dandelion

We should all be acquainted with what dandelions are, and the first to find out how to use them medically were the Native Americans. Did you know, for instance, that eating a dandelion salad (where you eat the leaves) will help relieve a sore throat? Do you also know the dandelion is a diuretic and can help you pass urine as a result? What you'll have to do is have some dandelion tea.

Smilax Bona-Nox

This herb has been used as a mild diuretic and a blood purifier. Used in the form of tea, this herb, using its roots, has also been used to cure arthritis. It can also help heal mild wounds, bruises, scrapes, and sores; the plant's leaves and bark should be mixed with lard. Sarsaparilla is from the genus

Smilax, a tropical herb. The growing, woody vine grows deep inside the rainforest canopy. It is native to South America, Jamaica, Mexico, Honduras, the Caribbean, and the West Indies.

Sarsaparilla drink

The common name of a soft drink popular in the early 1800s is also Sarsaparilla. As a home cure, the drink was used and was also served in bars. The sarsaparilla soft drink was normally made from another plant called sassafras, contrary to common opinion. It has been identified as being similar to root beer or birch beer in flavor. In some Southeast Asian countries, the drink is still popular but is no longer common in the US.

The benefits

Sarsaparilla produces a wealth of compounds from plants known to have a therapeutic impact on the human body. Chemicals such as saponins can help relieve pain in the joints and itching of the skin and kill bacteria. Other chemicals may be useful to minimize inflammation and to protect the liver from damage. It is important to remember that human experiments are either very old or absent from these claims.

Psoriasis

Decades earlier, the advantages of sarsaparilla root for treating psoriasis were recorded. One research showed that in persons with psoriasis, sarsaparilla healed skin lesions significantly. The researchers proposed that one of the key steroids of sarsaparilla, called sarsaponin, can bind to and extract from the body the endotoxins liable for the lesions in psoriasis patients.

Arthritis

A potent anti-inflammatory, Sarsaparilla is. This aspect also helps treat inflammatory disorders such as rheumatoid arthritis and other triggers of joint pain and gout-induced swelling.

Syphilis

Against toxic bacteria and other microorganisms that have infiltrated the body, Sarsaparilla has shown activity. It has been used for decades to cure major diseases such as leprosy and syphilis, but it does not work and present-day antibiotics and antifungals. Syphilis is a disease of sexual transmission caused by a bacterium. Another debilitating illness caused by bacteria is leprosy. In recent studies, the antimicrobial role of Sarsaparilla has been reported. One paper looked at the behavior of over 60 different sarsaparilla-isolated phenolic compounds. These compounds were tested by researchers against six kinds of bacteria and one fungus. The researchers reported 18 compounds having antimicrobial activity against the bacteria and one against the fungus, respectively.

Cancer

Recent research has shown that sarsaparilla has anti-cancer effects in multi-cancer cell lines in mice. Preclinical trials have also demonstrated the anti-tumor effects of sarsaparilla in breast cancer tumors and liver cancer. To discover that if sarsaparilla could be used in cancer prevention and care, further research is needed.

Protecting the liver

Sarsaparilla also showed beneficial effects on the liver. A study performed in liver-damaged rats showed that compounds abundant in sarsaparilla flavonoids could reverse liver damage and make it function at its best.

How to Eat

- The roots can be added to soups and stews.
- The young shoots can be consumed raw. They can also be cooked like asparagus.
- The berries can be consumed raw. They can also be cooked.
- The tendrils can also be consumed.
- It is generally used as an ingredient in soft drinks.

Curly Dock

Used as an ingredient in salads, curly dock is filled with good vitamins and minerals and has a sweet yet sour flavor. It is also a rich source of iron. It was often thought that the herb had laxative effects. The Cherokee mixed it with beeswax, a little oil, and ground it up. The salve has been used with mild burns, sores, rashes and other skin irritations as an ointment. Due to their tart, lemony taste, widespread availability, and the fact that they were free for the taking, docks were common wild edibles during the Great Depression. Today, this popular and tasty edible weed has been overlooked by most people. Docks are annual plants emerging from taproots, and they are most commonly found in open fields and along roadsides in neglected, disturbed soil.

Which Docks Are Edible?

There are several edible docks, but the most popular in the USA and Europe are curly docks and broad-leaved docks. Other docks that are edible have R. (Western dock) occidentalis, R. (yard dock) longifolius, and R. Stenphyllus stenphylus (field dock). R. In the American Southwest, hymenosepalus (wild rhubarb) is widespread in the desert. It is bigger than many other docks and is more succulent. For many Native American tribes, it has been a common source of food and dye.

Parts used for food

stems,Young leaves, seed.

Food uses of dock

They've tart, leaves tasting like lemon & are used in cooking similarly. Most young plants are always the finest to make a delicious 'spinach' while some find the flavor 'sour' yet 'hearty.' Use bacon, butter, eggs (hard-boiled) & seasoning to serve the greens. Like the vine leaves and rice, cheese filling and herb, the leaves may also be stuffed. Dried, they may be used for potatoes, rice, fish, or the sandwich spread as a seasoning. They produce vast amounts of fruits & nuts that can also be boiled into ground or mush to make bread, muffins and gravies & added to meal or flour. As a replacement for rhubarb pie, the young plants' stems could be sliced, simmered & sweetened with honey.

Nutritional profile of dock

The plants are also very nutritious. For instance, Curly Dock has far extra vitamin C compared to oranges and much extra vitamin A compared to carrots. This also contains B2 and B1vitamins& iron.

Dock recipes

Rice, Dock, seaweed parcelsand feta Cheese

Herbal medicine uses of dock

To soothe nettle stings, leaves are excellently used and sometimes grow near the offending plant. Calming properties were used for scalds, blisters and sprains, and have also been used for soothing stings and insect bites. They were a common treatment for staunching bleedings or blood purification. To cure wounds, the juice from leaves may be put in as a rub. The seeds were used to cure liver disorders, jaundice, skin conditions, constipation, boils, rheumatism, and diarrhea. The roots were used to cure coughs, colds and bronchitis.

3.6 Elderflower

In various ways, elderflower can be consumed: some of the most common are jelly, syrup, and tea. But be careful, for the flower section itself is the only edible component. Since they are poisonous, the leaves, roots, twigs and stems cannot be eaten safely.

What's used for medicinal purposes is the extract of the elderflower. The extract should, precisely, be used as a remedy for:Sweating

- Influenza
- The Common Cold
- Bleeding
- Bronchitis

- Constipation
- Colds

3.6 Flaxseed

To help heal the kidney, flaxseed has been used. It can also be used to relieve heart-related complications and sore throats. .As long as you don't eat it while it's raw or unripe, flaxseed can also be eaten in whatever way you see fit. The recommended way to use it is when it is in powdered form or dried form.

3.7 Lavender

Lavender could be the treatment you are searching for if you have suffered from any sleep-related issues. During a survival scenario, having plenty of sleep would be crucial to keep the energy levels up. To find it easy to sleep and calm the discomfort from headaches, the Native Americans will use the scent of lavender. It is extremely easy to make lavender oil. Steep the branches in olive oil (or water if you're in a condition of survival), and you'll be set.

3.7 Mint

Mint is well-known, even to those unfamiliar with herbal medicines. Besides being rich in magnesium, calcium, phosphate, and potassium, mint is safe because it is very high in Vitamin A and Vitamin C. To lower blood pressure and alleviate discomfort in the digestive tract, the Cherokee tribe will make mint tea. Crush the mint leaves to cure itchy spots and skin rashes, mix them with a little water to make an ointment and then rub the mixture directly to the infected region.

Mullein

For lung and respiratory issues, this traditional herb may help. The Cherokee burnt the mullein roots, inhaled the smoke they felt, opened the airways and relieved the mucous membrane's inflammation that lines the respiratory tract. For curing joint pain and migraine headaches, the flowers may be used to prepare a sedative drink. For asthma, whooping cough, measles, bronchitis, hoarseness, asthma, earaches, colds, chills, flu, swine flu, fever, nausea, sore throat, and tonsillitis, Mullein is used. Asthma, diarrhea, colic, stomach bleeding, migraines, knee pain, and gout are also found to be successfully treated with this herb. To improve urine production, it is also used as a diuretic. It is also used as a sedative. For cuts, bruises, burns, hemorrhoids, frostbite and skin infections, Mullein is applied to the skin (cellulitis). To soften and protect the skin, the leaves are used topically. In manufacturing, Mullein is used in alcoholic drinks as a flavoring component. Mullein is a respiratory tonic that is supreme, healthy and profound. It helps to open the lungs, relieves spasms, tightness and cough, and alleviates dryness and discomfort. In the garden, this common weed may be seeded. In lawns, meadows, and gardens, Mullein prefers the sunny, open, and disturbed soil. It is a biennial of self-seeding. This can move about from year. Throughout the season, harvest the happy-looking leaves for tea, sugar, steam, or tincture, but be cautious when spotting the plant before it flowers. Mullein has a slight fragrance and flavor. Make sure to strain the irritating hair through a paper filter.

About mullein oil

Mullein oil is derived from the plant's flowers or leaves. The oil is used for earaches, eczema, and many other skin disorders as a treatment. Based on a trial of 171 children aged 5 and 18 years old with an ear infection, one study showed some benefit for ear pain. With or without a topical anesthetic, they were given herbal drops or antibiotics. Researchers have discovered that herbal drops decrease discomfort. They also emphasized that they cost less than antibiotics and had no side effects.

Mullein oil two ways

Mullein oil can be produced by either cold (passive) or hot (active) processing from either dry or fresh parts of the plant.

Hot oil infusion

This method involves softly heating a carrier oil, like olive oil, with mullein leaves and/or flowers for up to three hours using a double boiler technique. Then it strains and stores the product.

Cold-steeped oil

For 7 to 10 days, the cold process typically involves steeping dried flowers and/or leaves in a carrier oil. Mullein oil is now widely available online and at

health food stores.

Benefits

Some active compounds of mullein include:

- saponins, that have pain-relieving, anti-inflammatory and antitumor properties
- flavonoids, that possess antioxidant as well as anti-inflammatory properties

- phenylethanoid glycosides, that have antioxidant, anti-inflammatory and antiviral properties
- iridoids, that possess anti-inflammatory properties

Antiviral properties

Verbascum species have been found to demonstrate antiviral activity against influenza A and herpes in several laboratory experiments. One laboratory research observed improved antiviral activity against influenza by mixing the drug amantadine with mullein. Mullein leaf is also sold in various forms:

- Tea
- Extract
- Oil
- Powder
- Capsule
- Elixir

Creams are often produced using the dried and raw forms (of the herb or flower). Some naturopathic practitioners and herbalists recommend mullein for curing inflammatory and respiratory issues, but there is not adequate clinical proof of its efficacy at present.

The takeaway

Herbal medicines can deliver real benefits, whether it is a relaxing tea or soothing balm. For thousands of years, Mullein has been around. For treating many problems, like cough and other respiratory conditions, its leaves and flowers have been used. It is available as tinctures, elixirs, tablets, and teas. With few reports of side effects, it's usually considered safe. For earaches and certain skin disorders, Mullein oil has been used.

3.8 Rosemary

Many Native American tribes knew Rosemary to be a holy herb, and with good reason: it is simply one of the most powerful natural plants for relieving joint and muscle pain. Rosemary will also help strengthen the immune system, the nervous system, indigestion, and circulatory system. It's one of the best plants you can get your hands on.

And all you've got to do is add that to the food. Rosemary has a warm plus bitter taste, and many foods offer a nice flavor and fragrance with this plant.

Moreover, it is possible to use Rosemary in tea or as an essential oil or liquid extract. Rosemary is famous for its flavor and smell; it is also recognized for the many health benefits it provides. For decades, Rosemary has been used for medical purposes as a healthy source of calcium, iron and vitamins A, C, and B-6.

Some of Rosemary's several possible health advantages include:

- Rosemary is a great source of vitamins as well as anti-inflammatory compounds that are known to help strengthen the immune system and increase circulation in the blood.

- Rosemary is known as a cognitive stimulant that can help to enhance the efficiency and performance of memory. Alertness, intellect, and concentration are all improved significantly by its use.

In people with persistent anxiety or stress hormone imbalances, rosemary aroma has been related to improving mood, calming the mind, and alleviating stress.

It has been effective in stimulating hair growth. Moreover, rosemary oil has been known to inhibit baldness, slow graying of hair, and cure dandruff and dry scalp.

For gastrointestinal disorders, including intestinal gas, heartburn, liver and gallbladder problems, and lack of appetite, rosemary is also used.

Rosemary is especially useful against bacterial infections. It is associated with staph infection prevention.

Rosemary nutrients help protect skin cells from damage frequently caused by sunshine and free radicals. Although research on rosemary tea and eye health is incomplete, evidence suggests that your eyes can benefit from some compounds in the tea. Animal tests have shown that it can delay the development of age-related eye diseases by incorporating rosemary extract into other oral therapies (AREDs). One research investigated the addition of rosemary extract to traditional therapies such as zinc oxide and other antioxidant combinations of AREDs, finding that it helped delay (AMD), a common vision-affecting disorder. Other animals and laboratory tests show that rosmarinic acid in rosemary prevents the onset of cataracts and lowers the occurrence of cataracts.

When consumed in low doses, rosemary is safe, but it can lead to severe side effects, like vomiting, spasms, or even pulmonary edema, when eaten in extremely high doses. Before adding rosemary into your diet, please check with your doctor.

How to make rosemary tea

It is very simple and easy to make rosemary tea at home. You only require two ingredients, i.e water and rosemary to make rosemary tea:

- Bring to a boil ten ounces of water (295 ml).
- Insert one tsp of loose rosemary leaves into the hot water. Then put the leaves in a tea infuser. Allow them to steep for five to ten minutes. This all depends on how tasteful you like your tea.
- Using a mesh strainer with small holes, strain the rosemary leaves from the hot water or remove them from the tea infuser. Used rosemary leaves should be discarded.
- Pour in a cup of your rosemary tea and enjoy. A sweetener, like sugar, honey, or agave syrup, can be added if you prefer.

Many remarkable health benefits are provided by rosemary tea. Your mood and brain, and eye health can benefit from drinking the tea or even simply inhaling its aroma. The oxidative disruption that may lead to multiple chronic disorders can also be avoided. It's necessary, though, to be mindful of its possible interactions with certain drugs. Using only two ingredients, rosemary tea can comfortably be made at home, and it fits perfectly into an overall safe and nutritious diet.

3.9 Sumac

The use of Sumac excellently achieves the cure of colds, fevers, and sore throats. You'll need to make sumac tea to get these advantages. Just pick and gently crush several berry clusters, soak them overnight in a pitcher of cold water, strain the mixture to extract the berries, and enjoy it. It's so easy. The discomfort is not going to go away absolutely, but you can feel almost instant relief, and that is better than nothing. In the Middle Eastern and Mediterranean cuisines, Sumac is a common ingredient.

In comparison, in herbal therapy procedures, individuals use it therapeutically. Sumac is a flowering shrub variety that belongs to a plant family known as the Anacardiaceae. Rhus coriaria is the scientific name. Cashew & mango plants are other common members of this genus. More than two hundred separate Sumac species have been identified, all of which belong to the Rhus genus. Though Syrian Sumac or Rhus coriaria is variety people cultivate most commonly for culinary use & herbal medicine. The big, thick clusters of pea-sized, bright red fruit it provides define Sumac. People could steep fresh fruits to make tea, but they dry them & powder more often for use as a herbal substitute or the culinary seasoning.

Potential benefits

The Sumac is common known as culinary spice. The People as well usedthis in cultural practices of herbal medicine for centuries.

It is rich in important nutrients

Sumac's complete nutrient profile is largely unclear, although little research suggests that it includes a host of beneficial nutrients. These include good fats, fiber, and certain important vitamins. A 2014 study showed that roughly 71 percent carbs, 19 percent fat, & 5 percent protein constitute nutritionally dried sumac. Two distinct types of fat, called oleic acid& linoleic acid, account for the fat's bulk in sumac. The type of monounsaturated fat typically associated with cardiac health is oleic acid. It is the primary fat present in other popular foods based on plants, including avocados and olives. Linoleic acid's a kind of vital polyunsaturated fat involved in the preservation of cell membranes and healthy skin. 2004 chemical study of fresh fruit of sumac showed that fiber, a nutrient that improves digestive health, makes up over 14 percent of it. Very little information is available on the correct micronutrient contents of the sumac, although several reports indicate that this contains a trace amount of some important nutrients, at least, including the vitamins B2, B1, C, and B6.

Rich in antioxidants

Multiple antioxidant mixtures are found abundantly in Sumac. Experts agree that this could be the primary explanation for the broad medicinal potential of Sumac. Antioxidants perform an important function to defend the cells from destruction & reduce the oxidative stress inside the body. There's also proof that antioxidants can play a role in reducing inflammation. They can help avoid inflammatory diseases, such as cancer and heart disease.

Facilitates balanced blood sugar

Some research suggests that sumac can be an important tool for treating blood sugars in people with Type 2 diabetes. A 2014 review of 41 individuals with diabetes examined the effect on blood sugar and antioxidant levels of a normal 3-gr dose of the sumac. At the end of the three-month trial, the normal blood sugar & antioxidant levels in the population consuming the sumac supplement were dramatically increased compared with those taking placebo. In another related report, forty-one people with diabetes were asked to take three grams of the sumac powder every day for three months. A 25 percent decrease in circulating the insulin was experienced by the sumac community, indicating that the insulin sensitivity might have improved substantially because of the sumac supplement.

Alleviates muscle pain

Research in 2016 gave a sumac drink or placebo to 40 healthy individuals to explore the sumac's ability to alleviate muscle pain. The group consuming sumac drinks reported substantially low exercise-based muscle pain at the end of the 4-week trial relative to the group receiving the placebo drink. Major changes in circulating the antioxidant levels were also seen in the sumac community. This might have induced the reported pain relief, the study authors proposed.

How to use

Sumac is a distinctive spice that can be used as herbal medicine or in food. Sumac is used most often by people as a seasoning. Sumac can increase the taste & color of several dishes, like many other culinary spices. It is especially common in the Middle East and Mediterranean households. Sumac has a rich red hue, a fragrance similar to citrus, and a distinct lemon juice-like tart taste. People often use it to make a sweet & sour drink called sumac lemonade. Sumac has a coarse, rough appearance when dried and ground. For many foods, namely grains, grilled meats & vegetables, baked goods, & sweets, ground sumac is excellent for adding acidity, clarity, and flavor.

Herbal supplements

As a herbal supplement, sumac is commercially available. Usually, people take this in capsule shape, but you may take this as tincture or tea as well. People dry these berries for use as a herbal remedy or culinary spice.

3.10 Yarrow

Yarrow is common worldwide and was first used by the Ancient Greeks to great effect, who used it by directly applying the leaves to stop excessive bleeding. They'd even take the yarrow juice and mix it with water as well. To better treat discomfort in the stomach or intestines, this paste would then be consumed directly. The Cherokee tribe was also well conscious of the potent medicinal properties of Yarrow, and they mainly prepared it as a tea, like the Ancient Greeks. To a cup of sugar, add a teaspoon of dried Yarrow, boil it for 10 minutes, strain the leaves and drink.

Moreover, to help cure dry skin, wrinkles, and open wounds, the Cherokee tribe would also spread Yarrow directly on the skin. Yarrow is a herb. Medicine is made with the above-ground components. Yarrow is used to curing flu, common cold, hay fever, menstrual absence, dysentery, diarrhea, lack of appetite, irritation of the gastrointestinal (GI) tract, and trigger sweating. To prevent toothaches, some people chew the fresh leaves. Yarrow is applied to the skin to stop hemorrhoid bleeding for wounds; and as a special bath for women with uncomfortable, lower vaginal, cramp-like problems. Yarrow can be used for bloating, intestinal gas (flatulence), moderate gastrointestinal (GI) cramping, and other GI symptoms associated with other herbs. Young leaves and yarrow flowers are used in salads. As a cosmetic cleanser and in snuff, Yarrow is sometimes used in manufacturing. In shampoos, yarrow oil is used. There are several chemicals in Yarrow that could affect blood pressure and could have anti-inflammatory effects. Significant quantities of Yarrow could delay the clotting of blood.

Uses and benefits of Yarrow Tea

Yarrow tea is made from a popular medicinal herb. For thousands of years, yarrow (Achillea millefolium) has been used because of its possible health benefits. In Greek mythology, the genus name, Achillea, alludes to the warrior Achilles, when he used yarrow to heal the wounds of his soldiers. There are 140 distinct species of Achillea, with clustered flowers and hairy plus aromatic leaves. Studies suggest that, as a herbal tea, extract, or essential oil, this plant can have multiple advantages. Here are a number of the basic advantages and uses of yarrow tea.

Improves wound healing

One animal study found that there were anti-inflammatory and antioxidant properties of yarrow leaf extracts, all of which aid wound healing. In addition, this study noted that fibroblasts, the cells responsible for regenerating connective tissue and helping the body heal from damage, can be enhanced by yarrow leaf extract. Meanwhile, a 2-week study of 140 women showed that an ointment made from this herb and St. John's wort helped treat episiotomy sites, which are surgical incisions made during childbirth on the vaginal wall.

Reduces digestive issues

Yarrow has long been used to relieve intestinal conditions such as ulcers and signs of irritable bowel syndrome (IBS), including pain in the gut, diarrhea, bloating and constipation. In fact, many flavonoids and alkaloids are found in this herb, that are plant compounds known to alleviate digestive complaints. A yarrow extract tonic defended against stomach acid damage in a study in rats and exhibited anti-ulcer abilities. Another animal study showed that yarrow tea's flavonoid antioxidants can reduce inflammation, digestive spasms and other symptoms of IBS.

Alleviates symptoms of depression and anxiety

Flavonoids and alkaloids can alleviate symptoms of depression and anxiety in yarrow tea. Studies suggest that plant-based alkaloids such as those present in yarrow tea decrease corticosterone secretion, a hormone that is high during chronic stress. One research showed that essential yarrow oils given orally to rats decreased anxiety and regularly promoted mental and physical activity.

May aid brain health

Many neurological conditions, such as multiple sclerosis, Alzheimer's, Parkinson's, and encephalomyelitis, inflammation of the brain and spinal cord triggered by a virus infection, have been seen to find support and cure from the use of yarrow. Recent animal research noted that the severity of encephalomyelitis and brain inflammation and spinal cord and brain injury caused by it were decreased by yarrow extract. Plus, a rat study showed that the antioxidants of yarrow had anti-seizure benefits, rendering this herb a potential therapy for epilepsy patients. Additional rat experiments suggest that Alzheimer's and Parkinson's disease signs, such as memory loss and physical movement deterioration and muscle tone, can be avoided by this plant.

May fight inflammation

Although inflammation is a normal response of the body, chronic inflammation can damage cells, tissues, and organs. Yarrow may minimize inflammation of the skin and liver, which can help cure skin diseases, indications of skin aging, and non-alcoholic liver disease. A test-tube analysis showed that yarrow extract reduced inflammation and increased moisture in the skin. Other test-tube experiments show that this extract can decrease inflammation of the liver and control fevers.

How to add it to your diet

Yarrow comes in a variety of forms, like tinctures, powders, ointments, extracts, and flowers and dried leaves. By steeping 1–2 teaspoons (5–10 grams) in boiling water for 5–10 minutes, the leaves and flowers can be made into tea. The dried herb and also premade tea bags can be purchased from different health stores or online. Yarrow powder can also be added to smoothies, water, and juice. Bear in mind that there is inadequate data to set dose standards for yarrow tea and other products. Before consuming this herb, you should still refer to product labeling and contact a healthcare practitioner.

From online or indifferent health shops, you can purchase dried yarrow or premade tea bags. It also comes in other types, such as tinctures, ointments, oils, and powders. Since ancient times, yarrow has been used medicinally, such as herbal tea. Research shows that wound healing, digestive problems, brain ailments, and other conditions can benefit from the plant compounds.

3.11 Basil

In the mint family, basil is a herb. It brings flavor to meals, and its nutrients can indeed offer health benefits. Basil is a delightful addition to soups, salads, and many Mediterranean dishes and is fragrant and simple to grow. The herb also provides oils and flavonoids that help protect the body from infection and disease. Basil has vitamin A, C and K, copper, manganese, calcium, iron, magnesium and omega-3 fatty acids that are beneficial. Basil can serve as an antiseptic for wounds and scrapes, as a healing herb, and it can give relief from headaches, flatulence, and loss of appetite. In a humid, sunny spot, grow your basil plant from seed, and keep the soil moist. An annual plant, basil is indeed very cold-sensitive. Cover it on days when the temperature drops to around 50 degrees. Snip the leaves for use. In many Mediterranean cuisines and particularly Italian ones, sweet basil (Ocimum basilicum) plays an important part. It forms a pesto base and adds to salads, spaghetti, pizza, and other dishes a distinctive taste. This herb is also featured in Indonesian, Thai and Vietnamese cuisine. Vitamins and a host of antioxidants can be provided by sweet basil in the diet. It has oil that may have therapeutic advantages as well. In several grocery stores, sweet basil is available, although other varieties have distinct tastes and fragrances. Tulsi, or sacred basil, is another form of basil (Ocimum sanctum). In Tamil and Ayurvedic medicines, which are mainly practiced in Southeast Asia, this plant plays a therapeutic role.

Health benefits

Basil consumption can help reduce oxidative stress. In the diet, as herbal medicine and as an essential oil, Basil can provide health benefits. Standard applications include, for example, the treatment of snakebites, colds, and irritation inside nasal passages, a frequent consequence of colds. Some macronutrients, such as calcium and vitamin K, are provided by Basil and several antioxidants. For instance, sweet Basil has a high concentration of eugenol, the chemical agent. This gives it a fragrance similar to clove. There are high concentrations of limonene in lime and lemon basil, which give them a citrusy scent. There are antioxidant properties of both eugenol and limonene.

Reduces oxidative stress

To remove free radicals from the body, antioxidants are necessary. Unstable molecules that form as a result of metabolism and other natural processes are free radicals. As a result of smoking and certain dietary choices, they may also grow. Compounds that help remove these molecules from the body are antioxidants. Oxidative stress can occur if they build up instead, resulting in cell damage and, potentially, disease. Scientists have linked oxidative stress to rheumatoid arthritis, cancer, heart disease, diabetes, and other health problems. The body produces some antioxidants, but it also needs to absorb some from the diet. Anthocyanins and beta carotene are among the many antioxidants that are found in basil

Supports liver health

A 2015 research in rats found that antioxidants had a positive effect on liver health in a powdered formulation that contained tulsi, or holy basil.

Fights cancer

A study released in 2013 examined whether cancer could be inhibited by tulsi or holy basil. The researchers concluded that some forms of skin, liver, oral, or lung cancers could be prevented by the phytochemicals found in holy basil. This is achieved by increased antioxidant function, modifying gene expression, galvanizing cell death and delaying cell division.

Guards against skin aging

Sweet basil has properties that could help protect the skin from certain effects of aging, according to studies published in 2011. In the analysis, a basil extract was applied by the researchers to laboratory skin models. The findings indicated that it could increase skin hydration and minimize roughness and wrinkling using basil extracts in topical skin creams. While basil extracts can affect some doses, the skin would not generally benefit from eating basil. However, if a person eats them as part of a varied diet, the antioxidants in basil and other plant-based foods may well have a protective impact.

Reduces high blood sugar

To better control blood sugar levels, some traditional medicine practitioners commonly prescribe basil. Research in rats in 2019 showed that an extract of sweet basil leaves helps lower elevated blood sugar levels. The findings have shown that basil leaves can help to treat high blood sugar in the long term. If further investigations verify these results, basil extracts may prove beneficial for people with diabetes.

Facilitates cardiovascular health

A 2011 study reported observations that a sweet basil extract lowered elevated blood pressure briefly, likely due to the extract's eugenol content. Eugenol can block the body's calcium channels, lowering elevated blood pressure. In another study, 24 healthy participants were given either a placebo or a 300 milligrams (mg) capsule of dried tulsi leaf extract once a day. Those who took the tulsi extract had lower cholesterol and triglyceride levels after four weeks compared to those who did not. The researchers concluded that the extract might help reduce some cardiovascular disease risk factors.

Boosts mental health

The formation of free radicals in the body is caused by mental stress. The plant contains properties that can benefit:

- Easing stress, depression, and anxiety
- Increasing the capacity to think and to reason
- Preventing memory loss due to age
- Enhancing stress-related sleep and sex disorders

Some research reported findings similar to those of diazepam and antidepressant medications. Confirming these observations, though, would take further research. Consuming tulsi, for example, in a drink, is also doubtful to have the same effect as receiving an extract dosage.

Reducing inflammation and swelling

Oxidative stress could exacerbate inflammation, a condition in various diseases, like Type 2 Diabetes, cancer and rheumatoid arthritis. Researchers analyzed the anti-inflammatory effects of two sweet basil essential oil formulations in 2017. Basil oil can help cure different diseases that include inflammation originating from oxidative stress, according to their findings.

Fights infection

Various traditional medicine practitioners have been using basil as an antimicrobial agent, and some scientific evidence confirms this use. Scientists added sweet basil oil to separate strains of Escherichia coli in 2013. The bacteria came from patients with infections of the respiratory, digestive, genital, or skin, and hospital appliances. The findings revealed that the oil against these bacteria was effective. The study determined that some basil oil formulations may help cure or avoid certain causes of infection.

Nutrition

According to the United States Department of Agriculture, the table below shows some of the nutrients in 1 tablespoon of fresh basil weighing around 2.6 g. It also shows how much of each nutrient an adult needs, according to **the** *2015–2020 Dietary Guidelines for Americans*. Keep in mind; however, that needs vary according to sex and age.

Tips for use

Basil is a fragrant herb with a distinctive flavor that many people enjoy. The various types have different flavors. In cooking, sweet basil is the most popular variety in the U.S., but people also use lemon basil, clove basil, cinnamon basil, and other types. A person could:

- Sprinkle fresh, chopped basil over a pizza or into a wrap.
- Arrange some basil leaves over slices of tomato and mozzarella, then drizzle the dish with olive oil.
- Add basil to soups, tomato sauces, and stir-fries.
- Make a marinade with basil, olive oil, and chopped garlic.
- Add whole, chopped, or torn fresh leaves to a salad.

Or, try these recipes:

- Chili chicken with fried basil
- Fresh basil pesto sauce
- Pasta with tomato and basil sauce

Native Plants for Native Medicine

As they have been for centuries, the same good healers are many of the plant remedies commonly available in pharmacies and natural food shops. Although many of us are acquainted with botanical immune boosters such as echinacea and elderberry, or witch hazel's skin-soothing ability (to mention only a few), numerous other plants have strong medicinal roots and are native to North America. Since ancient times, people have needed plants to improve their lives and make the act of living a little more comfortable, not just for their survival. Here are the powerful plants whose conventional uses continue to educate and influence how we care for our diseases and encourage human health.

4.1 California Poppy

It is possible to medicinally use all parts of the California poppy plant, from its bright orange roots to its leaves, flowers and seedpods. The flowers were prepared by the Costanoan tribe members as a strong tea to clean their hair and kill head lice. The seeds were ground by the Ohlone individuals and combined with bear fat as a hair tonic dressing. Tribes in Mendocino's region juiced the roots to cure several different illnesses, from headaches to stomachaches to toothaches. Moreover, nursing mothers would wash their breasts with root juice to help dry the milk flow when it was time to wean their babies. Pomo women made a poultice and/or a strong tea from the mashed seedpods and applied it for the same purpose to their breasts.

4.2 Gooseberry & Currants

Currants and gooseberries have long been used medicinally by indigenous people of North America. To soothe inflamed throats, the Comanche people used berry tea as a gargle. A decoction from the root was developed by the Prairie Potawatomi tribe, which was good eyewash to extract foreign particles or soothe sore or irritated eyes. The Muscogee (Creek) tribe drank a powerful tea produced from the root bark to remove intestinal worms. To soothe painful and inflamed skin tissue, gooseberry juice was often applied to the skin as a wash.

4.3 Milkweed

The latex juice from the milkweed stems, plant tops, and the stem has been used for medicinal purposes by many native tribes. The Miwok people used latex to cure warts. A decoction of the dried plant tops was made by the Cheyenne and used as an eyewash to treat snow blindness. Pleurisy root, also dubbed as butterfly milkweed (Asclepias tuberosa), was made into a cough remedy and was ultimately used by the people of Cherokee, Delaware, and Mohegan.

4.4 Nettles

The Hesquiaht and the Miwok people used the plant, often by whipping stems of fresh nettles over the infected body regions, to relieve muscle and joint pain. Transient burning and blistering were caused by the formic acid touching the skin, but it also generated a circulation rush to those parts. For problems such as arthritis, this increased circulation in the muscles and joints provided some permanent pain relief. Cherokee people and drunk prepared a tea from nettles as a stomach tonic. During gestation, the Cree Indians considered nettles an essential female herb.

4.5 Persimmon

Before the first frost, the Cherokee people gathered the fruits and turned them into an astringent herbal syrup to cure diarrhea.

The Choctaw sun-dried the fruit and, for the same reason, baked it into bread. The Catawba tribe developed a fruit poultice to cure warts and a decoction from the bark of the tree to use as a mouthwash for thrush (a type of fungal infection). To ease heartburn, the Rappahannock Indians used to chew the bark.

4.6 Spruce

In long, freezing winters, Native Americans knew that tea made from spruce needles helped people remain well. In Quebec City, Settlers started to suffer from scurvy in the 1500s (caused by a vitamin C deficiency). The Iroquois Indians shared with them this effective solution. In addition to curing them of scurvy, drinking spruce tea and spruce beer, dubbed Newfoundland spruce beer, became an essential preventive measure.

4.7 Willow

Along with many other tribes, the Choctaw and the Delaware Indians used peach leaf willow (S. amygdaloides) and other plants to make a toothbrush from a small willow twig.

Their teeth can be brushed, and the astringency of the tannins helped preserve good gums.

4.8 Yew

As a means of contraceptive, women of the Okanagan tribe and other northwestern coastal tribes consumed yew berries. To cure tuberculosis, arthritis and kidney failure, the Quinault people cooked the bark as a decoction and consumed it in very small quantities. The Cowlitz Indians developed a needle poultice and applied it to wounds topically. However, the leaves are not to be consumed orally since they are toxic.

Uses of Yew

In medicine and folklore, the yew has always occupied a special place. Being evergreen and renowned for its longevity, both death and immortality have been linked with it.

It has been recognized in the last decade that the pseudo alkaloids of different species of yew are effective antimitotic agents that are beneficial in some cancers that are highly resistant to other drugs. It is a slow-growing evergreen tree that can grow to 25 meters in height (80feet).

Its bark is rust-red, and the needle-like leaves are dark green. Paclitaxel is a drug extracted from the bark of the Pacific yew tree (Taxus brevifolia), the most well-known natural drug for the cure of cancer in the United States, and is used in the treatment of breast, prostate, and ovarian cancer, as well as Kaposi's sarcoma.

4.9 Chamomile

Another simple medicinal plant to grow at home is Chamomile that is quite popular as a soothing tea. Chamomile gives comfort to an irritated stomach, in addition to its soothing effects, which can relieve skin irritations. For decades, Chamomile has also been used as a soothing way to relax colicky infants. Chamomile plants like full sun and can grow to about 18 inches in height. It is easy to grow German Chamomile from seed.

Moreover, after the first season, the plants tend to self-sow freely. Within six weeks of planting, the beautiful daisy-like flowers emerge, supporting two plantings in one outdoor growing season. Cool, full sun and neutral climate favor German Chamomile in addition to mildly acidic, well-drained soil. Place the blooms to dry in a warm, dark place.

A common name for a large number of plants that look like daisies is Chamomile. To help people sleep and relax, these herbs have been used in the finest herbal teas. Chamomile contains coumarin, a drug that, much like aspirin, thins out the blood. This plant is indigenous to Europe and Asia but has now spread across the world. Native Americans have since been introduced to the plant, and they have immensely benefited from the plant. The plant holds substances that are so potent that pregnant women or women who are breast-feeding are advised against its use. Chamomile, since it has an anti-inflammatory effect, has also been as cosmetics. Did you know the Chamomile is also used for blonde hair enhancement?

Benefits of Chamomile

Chamomile is commonly used around the world and has many advantages and uses, as a muscle relaxant. This can assist with abdominal cramps, stomach pains, or muscle tension. Buy the herb and brew your tea. Many athletes have taken to chamomile following a tough workout to help calm the body. For most of the pains, two or three cups a day are adequate. The herb can also be used for the skin, and burns, asthma, and many other skin conditions can be healed. Chamomile has been used as a treatment for clearing acne and other skin irritations, as well as an anxiety remedy. The plant has oils that are very helpful to the human body, and its fragrance is popular. It has also been recognized that it is used to disinfect houses. To cope with digestive issues, as well as incense, the Native American herbal medicines used chamomile as a drink.

- Has many simple and stable applications
- Helps with headaches
- Nice to use with skin disorders
- Assists with cramps of all forms
- Has cosmetic features

Chamomile Uses

Chamomile may be used to produce tea, cream, or tablets for all sorts of other purposes. Tea can help with all types of things, primarily dealing with issues with the stomach. To cope with anxiety and heart attacks, numerous teas have been brewed with Chamomile. Chamomile has also been made into a cream that assists with issues with the scalp. You should apply the cream to help with bruises, wounds, as well as scrapes. The cream is also used for skin clearance, mostly for those with acne or eczema. Due to the oils, it contains, Chamomile has also been credited with minimizing unnecessary gas and bloating. It will help avoid a migraine before it even starts. Chamomile is a perfect treatment for migraines. Women who have had PMS or menstrual cramp issues will find chamomile tea a perfect and safe way to handle the said issues.

Pinyon

Pinyon is better known for its edible seeds. Although there are two pinyon species native to Utah, Colorado pinyon (Pinus edulis) and single-leaf pinyon (Pinus monophylla), Native Americans similarly use them. Pinyon has a broad range of medicinal applications. The pitch was used for various diseases, including wounds, some form of skin problem, digestive or intestinal disorders, infectious diseases such as colds, flu, tuberculosis, venereal disease, sore muscles, rheumatism, fevers, and internal parasites. It was also heated and subsequently applied to the face to remove excess hair or avoid sunburn. As an emergency ration, the inner bark was consumed or converted into an expectorant tea. To relieve fevers, the needles were chewed and swallowed to improve perspiration. To make a fumigant for earaches, buds were chewed and turned into a poultice for wounds or dried and pulverized. Making dyes or colors, gluing arrows, cementing turquoise jewelry, or waterproofing weaved water jugs or baskets were practical uses of the pitch. A tremendously important food source was pine nuts, and there were even more ways of consuming them than either raw or fried. They were mixed with berries and stored for winter use, made into cakes or gruel, mixed with yucca fruit pulp and made into a pudding, kneaded into seed butter, spread on bread, or made into hard dough, frozen, and eaten like ice cream. They may be ground into flour and rolled into balls. For added flavor, some tribes ground them with shells. Generally speaking, a strong pine nut harvest is only expected once every seven years. An outbreak of smallpox followed this, probably because several distinct groups gathered together to share the harvest and likely transmitted the disease. Practically every other aspect of the pinyon had used as well. Pollen has been used, often in place of cattail pollen, for ritual purposes. Since it was resistant to rot and wood-eating beetles, pinyon wood was valuable for house construction, and it was also used to produce useful things such as cradles, looms, saddle pieces, tools, and toys.

Juniper

Most of the medicinal uses of Juniper, unlike pinyon, were derived from infusions or boiling extracts of leaves, twigs, needles, or cones rather than from pitch. Nevertheless, with a list of disorders as long and variable, these preparations were used: renal complications, pneumonia, venereal disease, diabetes, cardiac problems, hemorrhages, stomachaches, vomiting, menstrual cramps, colds, fevers, smallpox, flu, cholera, tuberculosis, chickenpox, worms, swelling, rheumatism, burns, sore throats, hives or sores, and boils or slivers. To kill ticks on animals, a heavy decoction of the cones was also used. Bluish, berry-like cones with one or two seeds were boiled and eaten or dried and added to water for a drink or ground into a meal. They have been pierced and strung for beads as well. British Columbia's Okanagan-Colville tribe found the cones to be toxic and used them on bullets or arrowheads to kill people in warfare more easily, but they also made a drink from the cones and drank it in the sweathouse. Juniper bark served well as a torch. It was also well suited for storing fruit and covering floors, and thatching roofs for lining and covering pits. Juniper wood had many applications, as with other species, such as building lodges, corrals, fence posts, horse yokes, drums, flutes, spoked wheels used in a throwing game, bows, and bowls. The needles and boughs of Juniper had extra defensive powers over sickness, death, and sorcery. During epidemics, boughs were hanged around the house to keep away germs and were considered effective remedies to drive away bad spirits associated with death. For protection from grizzlies, hunters have even rubbed themselves with juniper boughs. For their holy, purifying smoke that could ward off disease, defend against ghosts, and eradicate the fear of thunder, the needles were burned ceremonially.

Douglas-fir

There were medicinal uses of all parts of Douglas-fir. Cuts, boils, other skin disorders, coughs or sore throats, including injured or dislocated bones, were cured by the pitch. It should be combined with oil and taken for abdominal discomfort, diarrhea, and rheumatism, among other illnesses, as an emetic (to induce vomiting) and purgative (a good laxative). It was also administered as a gonorrhea diuretic. The bark had antiseptic properties and helped with bleeding intestines and stomach, prolonged menstruation, and allergies induced by touching hemlock water. A strong general tonic and a remedy for paralysis are used through its needles. Bud tips for mouth sores are chewed. For colds, venereal disease, urinary disorders, or an emetic for high fevers and anemia, a decoction or infusion of young shoots was also used. Douglas-fir did not have as much fruit as some other trees, but the pitch could be chewed like gum or consumed as a sugar-like food, as in many other evergreens. The needles and young shoots could provide tea, and seeds were possibly used as a fruit, but they were not nearly as large and nutritious as the pinyon seeds. The wood found its way in such valuable tools as spear shafts, snowshoe frames, bows, tepee posts, and dugout canoes. Strong camping beds and sweathouse flooring were provided by Boughs. In basket making, twigs could serve as a coarse twine wrap, and pitch could be used for canoes as glue and patching material. To smoke buckskin, rotting wood was used, thereby retaining and dying it. For parts of the Douglas-fir, many tribes had separate ceremonial uses.

Ponderosa Pine

For sores and boils, aching backs and joints, sore eyes, earaches, and a general tonic, Ponderosa pine pitch was used medicinally. To speed up placenta delivery, hot needles were used, and a decoction was useful for coughs and fever. Boughs were used for muscle discomfort in sweathouses. To assist with hemorrhaging and high fevers, plant tops were used. Many tribes used the sweet inner bark for food. It could be eaten raw, rolled into balls for a tasty treat, baked into cakes, mixed with corn and meat and used to spice broth, or peeled off into strips and dried for later use as a highly nutritious food supply. It was obtained while the sap was running on cold, cloudy days, and various sources have compared the flavor to either sheep fat or lemon syrup. The seeds, either raw or fried, or dried and powdered and made into small cakes or bread, have also been used for food. Practical applications tended to outnumber the dietary and medicinal uses of ponderosa pine. The pitch can be used as a hair tonic, as a glue for the production of arrows and other items, and as a waterproofing agent for water jugs and moccasins. When out foraging, the bark was ideal for portable shelters or containers for sand painting pigments. The plentiful long needles could also be used to make baskets, insulate underground storage pits or pit house roofs, or provide a platform for roasting berries. A blue dye was produced using the roots, and the root fibers were used in basketry. The wood was useful for big roof timbers, fence posts, corrals, lodge sticks, dugout canoes, ladders, cradleboards, saddle components, and snowshoes.

Conclusion

The world cultures have concentrated and depended on conventional herbal medicine for centuries to fulfill their healthcare needs. The global market for herbal medicines is on the rise, amid the modern age's medical and technical advances. Currently, this sector is expected to gross over $60 billion annually. Some natural remedies can be more affordable and convenient than traditional medications, and since they comply with personal wellbeing principles, many individuals choose to use them. In their day-to-day life, Native Americans used a great number of herbs, and while most of these habits are no longer common, many ethnobotanical studies have introduced them to the world. While anthropologists have mainly concentrated on native applications of herbaceous and shrubby plants, various reports also show native uses of trees. Trees were used by Native Americans primarily for medicine, food, instruments, protection, and ritual aids. The needles of evergreens, for example, were widely used for tea.

Similarly, the pitch was chewed as gum, the inner bark was eaten for food and/or medicine, the wood was used for home and instrument building, and various parts were used for purification or cleansing. Similarly, the uses of these trees by various tribes vary considerably. Since ancient times, cultural health activities have been in place and continue to be essential means by which well-being is preserved and pursued. Traditional medicine is described by the WHO as the "total sum of knowledge, skills and practices based on theories, beliefs and experiences indigenous to different cultures, whether or not explainable, used in health maintenance along with in the avoidance, diagnosis, enhancement or treatment of physical and mental illness." The roots of Native American and Hispanic cultures are prominent in the Southwest, with traditional healing methods being common in both communities. Native American healing practices include herbal medicines to cure physical conditions; cleansing ceremonies in preparation for healing; and shamanism, based on the idea that spirits cause illness. Cultural healing techniques may be used by both Mexican Americans and Native Americans while still using Western medicine.

Nevertheless, you may wonder if herbal choices are safe. In a survival case, if you intend to use the herbs, learn to recognize them now so that you can identify them when you need them. If the Native Americans used them, maybe you too could use them safely and protect your life as a result.

CPSIA information can be obtained
at www.ICGtesting.com
Printed in the USA
LVHW052353141221
706194LV00011B/624

9 781914 107856